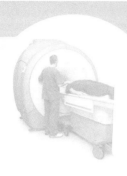

GW00480483

HELP!

SOMEONE I LOVE
HAS CANCER

Deborah Howard, RN, CHPN

Consulting Editor: Dr. Paul Tautges

© Day One Publications 2010

First printed 2010

ISBN 978-1-84625-217-4

All Scripture quotations, unless stated otherwise, are from the
English Standard Version (Crossway, 2001)

Published by Day One Publications
Ryelands Road, Leominster, HR6 8NZ

TEL 01568 613 740 FAX 01568 611 473

email—sales@dayone.co.uk

UK web site—www.dayone.co.uk

USA web site—www.dayonebookstore.com

Designed by **documen**
Printed by Orchard Press (Cheltenham) Ltd

To the hundreds of cancer patients
(and their families) whom God
has placed in my path as a
hospice nurse,
and for what they've taught me—
and to my beloved brother, John Koon,
who, in the way he transcended cancer,
served as a godly role model and guide.

Contents

ACKNOWLEDGMENTS

Thanks go to Paul Tautges, who introduced me to Day One Publications, for thinking of me for this project. Also:

To Judy Howe, my personal editor and lifelong friend.

To my "test" readers: Debbi Casey, Harold Goss, Theron Howard, Dr. Wayne Mack, and Curtis and Betty Thomas. Thanks for taking the time to read my work and tell me your thoughts.

To Dr. Reed Thompson, for fine-tuning the medical information.

And, as ever, to Theron, my husband and partner through life, who continually encourages me to keep writing. Thanks for sharing my ministry to comfort the hurting and encourage the fainthearted.

This volume will not answer all your questions about cancer. It is intended to be a primer—providing the basic information you, the loved one of a newly diagnosed patient, want and need to know. At the end of the book is a list of suggested materials and websites for more detailed information.

In this book, you'll find a definition of cancer and the way it forms, grows, and spreads, as well as descriptions of some of the more common treatment options. Since I am a certified hospice and palliative nurse and have worked with cancer patients for almost two decades, I can't resist the opportunity to also talk about the benefits hospice provides for terminally ill patients.

You'll find this book directed primarily to Christians—believers and followers of our Lord Jesus Christ. Though the *medical* information given applies to all, the *spiritual* reminders of the *promises of God* do not. The promises of Scripture to which I frequently refer are given to God's people alone.

With a heart that yearns for all to come to salvation in Jesus Christ, let me say a few words to non-Christian readers. Perhaps you've never seen the need for salvation. But the situation which has caused you to pick up this book may have made this a more relevant issue. To you I want to say that salvation doesn't depend on doing good works—or having our good deeds outweigh the bad. Romans 9:16 says,

> *It does not, therefore, depend on man's desire or effort, but on God's mercy.*
>
> (NIV)

Salvation is completely dependent on God!

You see, God is so holy that he cannot excuse sin. Even though, left to our own devices, we can come up with excuses that satisfy us, they will never satisfy his requirements. That's where Jesus comes in. He is our Sin-Bearer, our Savior. Though he had no sin, he took upon himself all the wretched sinfulness of all his people—past, present, and future. Then he died on the cross to pay the penalty for those sins so that his people could be considered righteous. In essence, he traded his "goodness" for our "badness," and our penalty was paid in full.

> And you, who were dead in your trespasses
> ... God made alive together with him, having
> forgiven us all our trespasses, by canceling
> the record of debt that stood against us with
> its legal demands. This he set aside, nailing it
> to the cross.
>
> (Colossians 2:13–14)

When he died on that cross, he did so as our substitute, taking upon himself the judgment we deserved. First Peter 3:18 reinforces this teaching:

> For Christ also suffered once for sins, the
> righteous for the unrighteous, that he might
> bring us to God, being put to death in the
> flesh but made alive in the spirit.

So Christ didn't remain on that cross forever, nor is he still in the tomb in which they laid him. Though we remember the cross and are eternally grateful for it, when we think of Christ, we need to understand that he defeated death, was resurrected, and ascended into heaven, where he sits at the right hand of God the Father. He secured victory for every one of his people, and it is because of his mercy that we can rest in that promised hope. And you could be one of those people for whom he died.

So the news is good! If we acknowledge our own sinfulness and inability to merit heaven, and cast ourselves on the mercy of God, he will redeem us through the blood of his Son, Jesus Christ. Christ trades his perfect righteousness for our sinfulness. It's only then that we can enter the kingdom free from the taint of sin—because he has removed our sinfulness and paid the penalty which belonged to us.

So I'm asking you, if you haven't done so already, to throw yourself on God's mercy. Ask him to deliver you. And he will! Romans 10:9 says,

> *... if you confess with your mouth that Jesus*
> *is Lord and believe in your heart that God*
> *raised him from the dead, you will be saved.*

It's a promise! It is my prayer that you will turn to him. Going through cancer is hard. Going through it without the hope that results from a relationship with Jesus Christ is horrible.

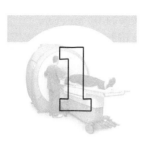

Let Me Walk with You

"I'm sorry, I don't think I caught that. I have what?"

"I said the tests are conclusive. You have cancer. I'm very sorry."

It doesn't matter what has transpired before we or our loved ones hear these words, or what happens after. In that first frozen moment, we tend to go completely numb. The impact is so great it paralyzes us emotionally—perhaps for months!

Our first response to disaster is disbelief: *No, that just can't be. Surely the tests are wrong. Maybe we need to see another doctor! This can't be happening to us.*

Maybe we're the ones receiving this diagnosis ourselves, or maybe those hateful words are directed instead to someone we love. Maybe that's worse.

A Page from My Own Story

I remember the day my brother, John, and I drove out to the neighborhood park. He wanted a beautiful, quiet place where we could talk.

John was forty-seven when he learned he had cancer. Through the next few years, he had chemo and radiation, remissions and recurrences. Each time the scans were repeated, we all prayed they would be clear.

However, on this day, almost four years after his original diagnosis, he quietly told me the results of his latest scans. They showed that not only had the tumors returned to his lungs, but more had appeared in other parts of his body. He simply said, "This is it, Deb."

Struggling to maintain my composure, I turned my gaze to my brother's face and saw an expression of total, quiet serenity.

I asked, "Are you really OK with this, John? Or are you just being brave for me? You don't have to put on an act. Not with me. Not ever."

He chuckled quietly, his blue eyes matching the sky's steel blue. Though my eyes brimmed with tears, his were clear and bright and even mirthful. Taking my hand, he said, "Let me explain something. If this news were about you, I don't know if I could handle it. But since it's about me, I'm fine with it. I'm in a win-win situation. If God grants me more time here, I win. But if he doesn't grant me that time, I still win. I know I'll be with Christ in heaven. That's the real victory. So I don't need to cry and scream and throw things. I really am fine with it. And the nearer I get, the more excited I am!"

That was the first time I realized that sometimes it's harder to walk this road with someone you love than it is to walk it yourself. If you are a believer, you have everything to look forward to after death!

That certainly doesn't mean that you won't grieve your own death. Some have a harder time with this than others. We need time to reflect upon our lives and ultimately to let them go. But the Christian facing death has nothing but marvelous joy and wonder ahead.

The perspective for the one who must find a way to say goodbye is a little different. To John, it ultimately meant being united with Christ, "going home." To me, it meant losing my brother. It meant going through life without him.

Besides, for millions, having cancer is *not* a death sentence. It's a time when their lives necessarily focus on treatment—their energies and efforts are directed to getting better. Their experience with cancer becomes a significant interlude in their lives. For those who beat the disease, life goes on.

My husband is an example of this. Diagnosed with prostate cancer in 2007, he opted for a prostatectomy. And, by the grace of God, he is now cancer-free. He suffered some slight discomfort, had a brief recovery period, and experienced some minor changes from the surgery, but it's basically back to life as usual for him.

However, as a hospice nurse, I haven't had many patients with such favorable outcomes. Instead, I've witnessed hundreds of families walking with their loved ones down the tortuous road toward the end of their lives, the same road I walked with John.

I've repeatedly witnessed the ways he and others triumphed over the disease. I've also seen the grace families have displayed while journeying with a loved one through the minefield cancer presents.

I pray this book will be relevant to the one who hears the diagnosis. But even more, I believe it to be relevant to their loved ones, the brave souls to whom I particularly write this book.

Is There No Escape in Sight?

The first step in this journey is to progress beyond denial. Denial is a monstrous foe that prevents constructive movement. It puts a barrier between you and God when that's the last thing you want! There should be nothing in your life or attitude to hinder your prayers to him.

When we're in denial, we deny the *providence of God*. We must remember that God is the divine Master-Planner of our lives. Nothing happens to us that is not brought about by his sovereignty and intended for his purposes. Death, sickness, heartbreak—all products of man's original fall in the Garden of Eden—are parts of his plan for us.

These elements of life are not given to us capriciously. They have nothing to do with chance or fate, but everything to do with the careful plan of a righteous and holy Father, who brings these things into our lives for a divine purpose.

It's natural for us to try to run from disaster. This is not new to our generation. King David eloquently described this particular kind of anguish in Psalm 55:4–7 when he wrote,

> My heart is in anguish within me;
>> the terrors of death have fallen upon me.
> Fear and trembling come upon me,
>> and horror overwhelms me.
> And I say, "Oh, that I had wings like a dove!
>> I would fly away and be at rest."

Most of us tend to try to escape pressure. We have other unattractive tendencies as well. We may want to whine, complain, lash out, or give up. However, the Scriptures tell us,

> Count it all joy, my brothers, when you meet trials of various kinds, for you know that the testing of your faith produces steadfastness. And let steadfastness have its full effect, that you may be perfect and complete, lacking in nothing.
>
> (James 1:2–4, emphasis added)

Meditate upon these truths. It's important for us to understand them, and to take them into our hearts and minds so we can apply them to the pressures we experience.

Another verse worthy of meditation in tough times is Isaiah 26:3, which says,

> *You keep him in perfect peace whose mind*
> *is stayed on you, because he trusts in you*
> *(emphasis added).*

Does "perfect peace" mean we're never tried or tested? No; but it means that we can be at peace in the midst of the trial.

Our earthly struggles should not come as a surprise to us. Remember 1 Peter 4:12:

> *Beloved, do not be surprised at the fiery*
> *trial when it comes upon you to test you, as*
> *though something strange were happening*
> *to you.*

Scripture shows that the Christian's life is typically peppered with suffering. In fact, we're promised hardship! Jesus tells us,

> *I have said these things to you, that in me*
> *you may have peace. In the world you will*
> *have tribulation. But take heart; I have*
> *overcome the world.*
>
> (John 16:33)

Thus, the Bible doesn't tell us that believers will not

suffer; instead, it assures us that we will! But it urges us to remain *steadfast* under the pressures of this earthly realm. What does it mean to be *steadfast*? We're told that when we remain steadfast, we will be made perfect and complete, spiritually mature and lacking nothing! Trials produce staying power and life transformation! Through trial, God molds us into the people he wants us to be:

> ... we rejoice in our sufferings, knowing that suffering produces endurance, and endurance produces character, and character produces hope, and hope does not put us to shame, because God's love has been poured into our hearts through the Holy Spirit who has been given to us.
>
> (Romans 5:3–5)

Suffering takes its toll on us, sometimes emotionally, sometimes spiritually—and sometimes physically. Sickness and death are a part of life. It is important that we look at our suffering through the lens of Scripture.

Thus, a cancer diagnosis doesn't mean that God has abandoned us. Cancer is not out of God's hands or bigger than he is; it is but another tool in his divine toolbox. Therefore, when we go through this kind of painful trial, it is important to constantly remind ourselves that our pain and suffering have a purpose!

We may not be able to see these results with our earthly eyes or conceive of them with our finite minds, but there is an overarching purpose to our lives—God's will, which is "good and acceptable and perfect" (Romans 12:2).

Our suffering will always produce two results—good for us and glory for God. Always!

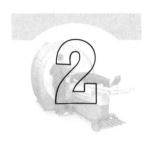

Knowledge Is Power

When devastation strikes, our first impulse may be to run from it. Instead, we need to hold fast to the Scriptures and stand firm under the pressure of our tribulations. So how can we stand firm while moving beyond denial?

The answer is simple though the task itself can be tough. First, you must ask yourself if you could be in denial. Ask God to help you see the situation clearly and to give you the strength and wisdom to handle it. After that, take a realistic look at your situation, learning all you can about it (its physical, emotional and spiritual aspects). Soon you'll be able to replace pretending [unreality] with fact. In that way, you can move past the paralysis of denial to acceptance of the task at hand ... It

is only then, when you are grounded in reality,
that you can truly be an effective help and
comfort for someone who needs you.[1]

Therefore, one of the most effective ways to move beyond denial is education. When a commander develops his plan for an upcoming battle, he wants to know his enemy's strengths, locations, and formations. He understands how they've operated in the past so he can more accurately predict their future moves and plan a strategy to defeat them.

We must do the same with cancer. Knowledge is power over this enemy. We need to know how strong it is, where it's located, and where it seems to be going. We need to comprehend the way it's behaved in the past to be able to anticipate what will happen next.

Make yourself an expert on your loved one's specific type of cancer. Cancers do not behave alike. Some are fast growing; others are slow growing. Some spread quickly; others don't. Some have high cure rates; others ... well, they don't. So learn about it. Read. Talk to people who have been through it. Go to doctors' appointments with your loved one whenever

1 Deborah Howard, *Sunsets: Reflections for Life's Final Journey* (Wheaton, IL: Crossway, 2005), 29.

possible. Ask questions. The more you understand, the better you'll be able to confront the disease. If you're familiar with its usual course, you'll be in a better position to make decisions about selecting or refusing treatment.

What Is Cancer?

This book is not designed to tackle all the intricacies of cancer. Cancer research is producing results and information at an astounding rate. Even oncologists (cancer specialists) are learning something new about it every day. But the following is a general overview of this complex disease.

Cancer is any of a group of diseases involving the unrestrained growth of abnormal cells in the body. It can form in almost any organ or tissue, even the bone marrow, where blood cells are formed.

Normal cells somehow mutate (change) into abnormal ones. Once these abnormal cells are produced, they rapidly reproduce themselves. A grouping of these cells forms into what is commonly called a *tumor*, starting very small and usually growing at an ever-accelerating rate.

These cells grow and divide more quickly than most normal cells and show a lack of differentiation, which simply means that they stop acting like the normal cells around them. For instance, heart cells have a certain function, and all the cells in the heart behave in such a way that this function is carried out. Similarly, other cells act in such a way that their own function is carried out.

Cancer is said to be a *progressive* disease because these abnormal cells accumulate until the cells begin to cause the organ to act contrary to its original function and design. Tumors are a little like parasites—useless to the body, yet consuming the body's nutrients (one reason why many cancer victims experience significant weight loss).

Cancer Warning Signs

The range of symptoms associated with cancer is vast and varied. Symptoms depend on the location of the cancer, the type of tissue, and the extent of tumor growth. The following is a list of the most common symptoms of cancer. Any one of these symptoms could be a warning sign of cancer and would need to be investigated.

▶ Rapid, unexplained weight loss.

▶ A scab, sore, or ulcer that doesn't heal within

about three weeks.

▶ A blemish or mole that changes in size, shape, and/or color, and which may bleed or itch.

▶ Severe recurrent headaches.

▶ Difficulty swallowing.

▶ Hoarseness that doesn't resolve within a week or so.

▶ Coughing or bloody sputum.

▶ Persistent abdominal pain or tenderness.

▶ Change in the shape or size of the testes.

▶ Blood in the urine without pain upon urination.

▶ Change in bowel patterns.

▶ Rash upon or bleeding/discharge from the nipples.

▶ Lump or change in shape of breast(s).

▶ Vaginal bleeding or spotting between periods or after menopause.

▶ Unexplained or nagging pain that doesn't resolve within two or three weeks.

Cancer Stages

The concept of the stages of cancer is important because treatment and survival are directly related to the stage of cancer at the time of diagnosis. Those involved with cancer patients soon hear statements such as, "It's progressed to Stage IV now," or, "The doctor says it's still Stage I." What does that mean?

In general, stages of cancer are from Stage O to Stage IV.

- *Stage O* refers to *carcinoma in situ*. These are lesions the doctor may refer to as "precancerous." They are usually superficial and don't typically collect to form an invasive tumor.

- *Stage I* refers to generally small tumors localized to a single part of the body.

- *Stage II* refers to larger, more advanced tumors, but still localized to one part of the body.

- *Stage III* is locally advanced, but has spread to regional lymph nodes.

- *Stage IV* refers to cancer that has spread outside its original site to another part of the body. This is referred to as *metastatic cancer*.

The spread of cancer from its original site to another is called *metastasis*. Cancer spreads through the lymphatic system, the bloodstream, or invasion into neighboring tissue. These cancer cells form new, satellite tumors which independently begin their growth cycle in their new site. Therefore, if you hear the term "metastatic lung cancer," it means lung cancer that has spread to another part of the body.

One thing few people realize is that if, say, lung cancer spreads to the brain, it does not become brain cancer; it's lung cancer in the brain. Thus, if prostate cancer spreads to the bone, it is not bone cancer; it is prostate cancer in the bone, and so on.

Malignant tumors are different from *benign* tumors. Malignant tumors are cancerous, grow rapidly, and have the propensity to invade and disrupt normal tissues and to spread. Benign tumors are non-cancerous and self-limited. They do not usually spread and are not, in and of themselves, harmful. And, though there are exceptions, they are not considered dangerous and require little or no treatment.

Outlook

I know there are millions who have beaten the disease. Today, almost half of all cancers can be cured completely. And both cure and survival rates continue to improve. Cancer is no longer considered a hopeless disease.

As a hospice nurse, however, I rarely see these success stories where patients are cured and go on to lead healthy, happy lives. My patients have exhausted all treatment options and the cancer continues to grow. Nevertheless, I have seen scores of "success stories." These patients may not have beaten cancer, but they managed to live their lives to the end with quiet joy and grace.

No Substitute for Prayer

As I said earlier, knowledge helps; yet it is no substitute for prayer.

God is our sovereign Master. It is by his hand that both blessing and calamity are brought into our lives. Therefore, he is the only true Cure. It is by his grace that we are healed, and it is also by his grace that we aren't.

When heartbreak occurs in your life, don't think

that he is unmoved by your pain. He is our present help in time of trouble. He is our Comforter and Protector. Our suffering is given to us for specific reasons, customized to each one of us. Relief from that suffering occurs only after those purposes are accomplished. But we're told to go to him with all our burdens. We are to cast our cares upon him. Our Father is compassionate and loves us more than anyone else ever could!

Faith is important all the time. Yet most of us would prefer lives that don't require it! If we were ordering our own lives, how many would ordain for ourselves the painful trials that make us stronger? It is important for us to realize that God does things we cannot comprehend.

> For my thoughts are not your thoughts,
>   neither are your ways my ways, declares
>   the LORD.
> For as the heavens are higher than the earth,
>   so are my ways higher than your ways
>   and my thoughts than your thoughts ...
>   (Isaiah 55:8–9)

No, there is no magic formula that will get our wishes and hopes granted. God is not a genie in a bottle, waiting to carry out our every command. He's our Master. We are dependent on him for everything. So we must throw ourselves upon his mercy, and trust that he will do what is best for us *every single time*. It may not feel like it when we're hurting, but it's true.

> And we know that in all things God works
> for the good of those who love him, who have
> been called according to his purpose.
> (Romans 8:28, NIV)

That's a promise. And "all things" encompasses everything—including cancer.

So go to your Father in prayer. Then leave your petitions in his care, knowing that he will compassionately give you exactly what you need in its proper time.

It all boils down to *trust*.

> As hard as it is to do sometimes, our
> responsibility as children of the Father is
> merely to trust Him ...
>
> Why should we trust Him ... ? Because of who
> He is! Because He commands us to. Because

29

*He has repeatedly shown us He is worthy
of trust. He is all-powerful and almighty
yet all-loving and compassionate. He is
completely faithful even when we are not. He
is completely reliable even though we falter.
He loves us in every situation and promises to
wield His power to fulfill His purposes in ways
that will ultimately benefit us and bring glory
to His Name.*

*We may not like what He brings our way, but
through it all we are asked to trust Him.*[2]

2 Deborah Howard, *Where is God in All of This?*
   (Phillipsburg, NJ: P&R, 2009), 151–152.

What Are
the Options?

Once you've escaped the numbness of denial and educated yourself about your loved one's cancer, what comes next? How do you move beyond the reality of the illness and the knowledge of how it behaves?

The following is a brief overview of the options available to those who've been diagnosed with cancer.

1. Chemotherapy

The purpose of the *chemo* is either to kill the tumor cells or to stop them multiplying. Chemotherapy may be given in pill form or topically, but the most common method is intravenous infusion. If chemotherapy is recommended, it can usually be accomplished on an outpatient basis. The schedules vary widely. The oncologist will come up with a specific drug regimen and treatment schedule tailored to your loved one's particular cancer.

Chemotherapy requires a delicate balancing act. The chemotherapy drug is selected according to its effect on specific cancers. Think of it as a poison designed to kill cancer cells. The oncologist must give the patient enough to kill those cells without giving so much that it begins to harm normal cells, particularly blood cells. So it is important for the oncologist to keep up with each patient's blood count before chemo is given. In most cases, blood is drawn and sent to the lab to be tested before each session.

The problem with chemo is that it is designed to attack rapidly dividing cells—and cancer cells usually divide very rapidly. But so do other cells in the body, such as those in the bone marrow, the intestinal lining, and the hair follicles (explaining the baldness that often accompanies chemo), or inside the mouth (hence the painful mouth sores that can occur).

For these reasons, chemotherapy patients are usually given prophylactic drugs before their dose of chemo. These medications are designed to offset some of the more unpleasant side effects of the powerful drugs—such as fatigue or severe vomiting.

People respond in different ways to the chemo.

Your loved one's particular dose or drug regimen is tweaked this way or that depending upon how the cancer responds to the drug and how well the patient tolerates the side effects.

2. Radiation

If radiation therapy is needed, the patient generally undergoes treatments several times per week, typically given on an outpatient basis. The treatments are designed to penetrate the body's tissues to an exact location where the beams of radiation are focused. They destroy or slow the growth of abnormal cells in the pinpointed area.

With today's sophisticated equipment, radiation rarely causes damage to normal cells. Cure rates depend upon how early the cancer has been detected, the location of the growth, or the specific type of cancer. In most cases, the treatments are painless and take only a few minutes.

In certain cases, *radiation seeding* is utilized. In this treatment, tiny pellets of radiation are implanted inside the tumor, where the abnormal cells are destroyed from within instead of from outside the body. This treatment is especially used for prostate cancer or pituitary tumors.

In some cases, radiation is the therapy used to try to destroy or shrink the actual tumor. In other cases, surgery may be performed to remove the tumor and radiation is prescribed to destroy any remaining abnormal cells that might have been missed by the surgery.

In cases where the cancer has advanced too far to expect a cure, radiation can be a tool in palliative (comfort) care. It is sometimes used to shrink a growth that is causing substantial pain but cannot be removed or destroyed completely; in these cases it is thought of as a *comfort* measure rather than a *curative* measure.

Some of the more unpleasant side effects possible with radiation include fatigue, nausea and/or vomiting, loss of hair, and reddening and/or blistering of the skin; all of these are usually temporary.

3. Surgery

When the tumor is still at Stage O–III and is therefore localized to one area of the body, surgery is often a viable option. A surgeon will remove the tumor and the surrounding tissues, sending multiple tissue samples to the lab to make sure that all the abnormal cells are gone and only healthy tissue remains. When the surgeon gets the "all clear" from the lab, he closes the incision and sends the patient to the recovery room. If necessary, the patient will be referred to an oncologist for preventive chemo and/or radiation to make sure all the cancer cells have been destroyed. Other times, when the surgeon believes all the cancerous tissue has been removed, there is no need for follow-up chemo or radiation.

If the cancer has advanced to Stage IV, the patient is usually no longer a surgical candidate (though surgery may be recommended, even in Stage IV, if needed to help relieve a troubling symptom). Once the cancer has spread beyond its original site, it becomes fruitless to try to remove only a portion of it. There are also cases when an exploratory surgery is performed but the cancer is so extensive that the surgeon determines it to be of no use to try to remove it.

4. Hospice

At the point when the doctor tells a patient that nothing more can be done medically, and no cure can be expected, many people turn to hospice to manage their care for the remainder of their lives. Others, for various reasons, opt for hospice from the time of original diagnosis and bypass all treatments aimed at controlling the cancer.

As I've already mentioned, millions have survived cancer. They have survived it by God's grace, having utilized some of the therapies mentioned above. I believe also that some occasionally experience miraculous healing of their cancer. If they have survived cancer by any means, that's wonderful! But what about those who don't have that kind of desirable outcome? What about those whose hearts are breaking because someone they love is about to be taken from them?

In this section I want to describe the practicalities and graces of hospice care. Please don't see this as a discouragement, but as an encouragement to those who are taking their first steps along this difficult journey.

Which option you and your loved one choose is a very personal decision. These choices are often fraught with misinformation and worry about the unknown and the "what if"s. Therefore, it is important to dispel some of these myths and to provide instruction and support regarding the path that lies ahead for terminal cancer patients and their families.

Whenever people call to ask my opinion about

their treatment options, I tell them I can't make the decision for them. But I *can* inform them of the benefits and risks of their options so they can make better, more educated decisions for themselves. At times like this, they need a clear understanding of such things. Given their specific situations and preferences, they take the information they've acquired (not just from me but from all other resources), decide if the risks outweigh any potential benefits, and choose the options that are right for them.

Those who want to continue to fight their illnesses with everything they've got need to ask their doctors one question: "What is the goal of treatment for me?" If the answer is that there is a good probability of an actual cure, I say, "You've got to go for it!" Otherwise, you might find yourself questioning your decision and wondering, "What if ...?"

For others, it's not so certain. It's true that one option is chemotherapy and others are radiation or surgery. Some travel to cancer centers that specialize in their type of cancer. Some use diet and natural remedies to fight their disease. As those walking beside our sick loved ones, we must support whatever they choose to do.

However, our loved ones may choose another way—

that of refusing further treatment. If the answer to your question regarding the goal of treatment is "To prolong the inevitable," you might be among those who choose no curative treatment at all. Some of my hospice patients have decided upon this option. They tell me they have decided to "let nature take its course."

Others come to hospice after exhausting all curative treatments. Most tell me that without the chemo and radiation, they actually feel better. Both groups know they might not live as long as they would if they sought or continued aggressive treatment, but often the time remaining for them is sweeter, healthier, and more satisfying once they've opted not to receive further treatment for their cancer. They will, of course, continue to receive treatment for comfort.

Among those who might choose the option not to seek curative treatment are the elderly, who often have multiple health problems. They are sometimes so fatigued with the struggles of life or other illnesses that they choose to enjoy life as long as they can without treatment.

Sometimes I see family members trying to get their loved ones to change their minds—urging them to get the chemo or the radiation the doctor recommends. All I ask is that we should keep in mind that those who choose no treatment deserve the same support and respect as those who choose aggressive treatments.

Still, many are afraid of hospice. They don't know if hospice is right for them because they don't understand what it's all about.

What do I mean by the term "hospice"? Hospice is an organization made up of professional people (doctors, nurses, aides, social workers, and counselors) with the common goal of managing the care of those with a terminal disease. Its focus is on providing comfort to the dying and support to the families. Hospice workers see patients anywhere they live. They can have hospice care at home, in a nursing-home facility, in the hospital, or in a hospice inpatient facility.

When talking to patients and their families, I sometimes hear that the patient's reluctance to participate in hospice is because he or she is holding out for a miracle. The patient might even believe we are trying to take away his or her hope by suggesting hospice.

In such cases, I offer reassurance that we will join the patient in prayerfully looking for a miraculous cure. There is no need to *plan* for a miracle. If one occurs, the patient is happily discharged from hospice care and goes back to his or her life with renewed joy and praise for God.

However, there *is* a definite need for planning if the miracle does not occur. And that's where a hospice program shines—in the medical management of the disease, assisting families in caring for their loved ones, and helping them come to terms with loss as the end of life looms closer.

Another misconception is that you have to be on your deathbed to qualify for hospice. Not at all. In fact, many of our patients are able to travel, garden, work, and enjoy life for quite a while before the disease starts limiting their activities.

We have a saying in hospice, "We know we cannot add days to your life, so we try to add life to your days." We may not be able to stop the inevitable, but, in most cases, we can ensure a calm and peaceful death by careful management of the symptoms that occur at the end of life, by instructing and supporting the family, and by providing a safe and comfortable environment for the dying person.

What benefits does hospice provide? Many!

▶ Perhaps most importantly, we ensure that the patient and the family will not have to walk this road alone.

- Hospice patients benefit from our experience.

- Hospice patients have a direct line to a nurse at all times. And the nurse has a direct line to the hospice doctor at all times.

- Each patient has a certified nursing assistant who helps with hygiene and safety.

- Each patient also has access to a social worker, a chaplain, a volunteer, and, in most cases, a bereavement counselor.

- Hospice patients no longer have to endure the hardships of doctor visits and hospitalizations. Except for heroic measures (ventilator support, defibrillation, blood transfusions, etc.), hospice can do everything in the home that can be done in a hospital.

Hospice does not take over a patient's care, but continually trains families to care for the patients more proficiently, with as little stress as possible. We want to take care of the caregivers!

I've covered a few important issues you need to know. Other important issues regarding cancer progression will need to be understood and discussed so that responsible decisions can be made. Such issues include artificial hydration and nutrition, signs and symptoms of impending death, maximizing your loved one's comfort, and other matters related to preparing for approaching death.

I don't believe that these issues should be dealt with in this kind of book. Some information should be gathered along the way, not at the outset of the journey. In a previous book, *Sunsets: Reflections for Life's Final Journey*, I dealt with these matters in more detail. That book may be helpful to readers who are ready to tackle these tough issues.

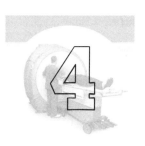

When I Am Afraid,
I Will Trust God

This is hard stuff, isn't it? I've been through these issues hundreds of times and they still weigh heavily upon my heart. And once, as I've mentioned earlier, I went through this with someone I dearly loved.

My brother, John, proved to be an amazing example of how to experience this journey with grace and joy—keeping a godly perspective and attitude every step of the way. What did he do that exemplified the proper attitude? And more than that, what standard does God use to show us the way during the hard times? I hope these next sections serve to answer those questions.

Where Do We Go from Here?

I keep referring to John because I love to remember him. But more than that, I want you to understand that I'm not accepting an impersonal writing assignment, pounding away at a keyboard from some lofty place where pain and suffering can't reach me. I have shared this pilgrimage with you.

My heart has been broken many times because of cancer—not only by John's death but also by losing countless patients and friends to cancer. And after all that, I don't have it all figured out. Nobody does! But, through my hospice experience, I have learned some things that may prove helpful to others. That's why I agreed to write this book.

I know this illness is scary and fraught with difficult decisions. Yet we need not be afraid. One helpful verse of Scripture I lean upon is,

> When I am afraid,
>   I put my trust in you.
> In God, whose word I praise,
>   in God I trust; I shall not be afraid.
>   (Psalm 56:3–4)

King David was in a potentially deadly situation when he wrote those words. Yet he trusted fully in the One he knew was over all things.

Jesus Christ provided the perfect example for us to follow, setting the standard for all believers. When he suffered horribly to pay the price for our sins, he demonstrated how we are to respond. First Peter 2:23 says,

> *When he was reviled, he did not revile*
> *in return; when he suffered, he did not*
> *threaten, but* continued entrusting himself
> to him who judges justly *[God the Father]*
> (emphasis added).

Jesus Christ, who had all power and could easily have escaped this ultimate suffering, did not do so. Instead, he entrusted himself to God. Should we do any less? Even through the happy, healthy years, we must continually entrust our lives—as well as the lives of those we love—to God, who makes no mistakes. It's vitally important to remember to trust him in all things—including our present circumstances.

Where Is God in All This?

Knowledge is power—I have already asserted that fact. It's important to understand all you can about cancer, but it's even more important to comprehend where God fits into all of this. What you believe about that determines, to a large degree, how well you will take this walk for yourself, how well you will be able to walk it with your loved one, and how you will live the rest of your life.

God doesn't fit into some little cubby-hole in our lives. Instead, he fills and determines every part of our existence, whether we acknowledge it or not! When, in our finite minds, we relegate God to a cubby-hole, gathering dust and ignored, we supplant him in our hearts with a counterfeit! We become the gods of our own universe! That's a dangerous thing to do. God describes this as a characteristic of the wicked!

> *In his pride the wicked does not seek*
> *him [God];*
> *   in all his thoughts there is no room*
> *   for God.*
>
> (Psalm 10:4, NIV)

Is there room for God in your life?

It's an understatement to say that God doesn't like it when we set ourselves up as our own gods—laughable reflections of our own ignorance. He makes it very clear that he is God and we belong to him. Here are some examples:

> I am the LORD your God ... You shall have no other gods before me.
>
> (Exodus 20:2–3)

> ... for I am God, and there is no other;
>   I am God, and there is none like me,
> declaring the end from the beginning
>   and from ancient times things not
>   yet done,
> saying, "My counsel shall stand,
>   and I will accomplish all my purpose."
>
> (Isaiah 46:9–10)

The sad truth is that we need constant reminders that he is God and we are his servants. A more fitting term is "slaves." If we belong to the Lord, we are his slaves—a joyous bondage in which we have the privilege to worship and serve the One who made us in the first place, One whose love for us is greater than any mortal heart could muster or imagine!

Sometimes, it takes trial and tribulation to remind us of who we are and who he is. And sadly, some people only pray when they're desperate! Let's not be like them.

It is in the midst of suffering that we fully recognize our helplessness and God's power. When we realize that truth, we can then turn to him for the answers to the problems that assail us. When we remember that only he can turn the tide of events that cause us pain, our prayers become fervent pleas instead of halfhearted requests.

As I said earlier, during these hardships, we must remember that God is not a genie in a bottle, waiting around to grant our every whim, but he is the great Jehovah God, the Maker of the heavens and the earth! What is important is that *his* will be done and not our own. He is God! He is so big and so infinitely intelligent that he makes decisions we cannot comprehend.

God is involved in every aspect of our lives: where we live, whom we love, what we do for a living, what our strengths and weaknesses are, whether we are healthy or whether we're not.

In any case, we are to honor God by seeking to live lives pleasing to him—not the other way around. Our whole existence should reflect this overarching desire to please and serve him. We must view our lives through that spiritual lens. In regard to every aspect of our being, we should ask, "How can I best serve him through this?"

Did you just lose your job? How can you love, serve, and please him through that? Have you been wounded by someone you considered your friend? How can you love, serve, and please him through that?

Did someone you love develop cancer? How in the world can you honor God, serve him, love him, and please him in relation to this kind of bombshell blowing your life apart? Is it even possible to do this?

Yes. It is not only possible, but God commands it! He charges us to trust him in everything! We are to view everything in our lives as being in his domain. The obstacles he places in our path are *designed* to result in our good and in his glory.

> ... *call upon me in the day of trouble;*
>   *I will deliver you, and you shall glorify me.*
>   (Psalm 50:15)

Does deliverance always take the form of making the bad stuff go away? No. Does it mean that God will grant you a miracle? No, though he might. Deliverance actually means that God will guide you through every hardship, even when death awaits you at the end. He is a refuge, a fortress, a haven.

We can always rest in his love. I find great comfort in the verse which says,

> *He will cover you with his feathers,*
>   *and under his wings you will find refuge;*
> *his faithfulness will be your shield and*
>   *rampart [fortification].*
>
> (Psalm 91:4, NIV)

It's such a visual verse and gives me much relief when I feel I need a safe place to rest, protected by his strength and faithfulness.

Yes, it glorifies God when we submit our wills to his. Humble submission pleases him, and demonstrates our love for him and trust in him in the midst of every trial. But that particular state of grace cannot be generated by our own sinful hearts. God knows it is impossible for us to submit in and of ourselves. He must give us the grace to do so. *He* supplies the kind of faith and strength that equips us to find such an *un*earthly attitude reigning in our hearts when we drop to our knees to say, "Oh, Lord

Jesus, I don't understand why this is happening, but I know that it is by your hand of providence that this has been placed in my life. I throw myself upon your mercy and ask that you give me whatever I need to honor you through this situation. Help me to have an attitude of sweet submission, Lord. Not *my* will but *yours* be done."

We are to pour out our concerns before him, then trust him to answer our prayers *in the way he sees fit*. Many times I've pictured dropping my troubles before God and saying, "OK, here they are. Do with them whatever you deem best."

The tricky part is that you have to actually mean it! When we come to a place where we fully trust the Lord *in everything*, then we feel we can truly let go of our own desires and live to obey his. We must develop absolute confidence in the fact that his will is the best thing for us, whether we agree or not, whether we understand or not. He gives us what we need at just the right time.

In the realm of cancer, we must understand that whether he chooses to bring healing to our loved ones or chooses to use cancer as the tool to end their earthly struggle, God is on his throne and always wields his power thoughtfully, perfectly, and lovingly to his children.

The truth is that people die. As Isaiah 40:6b–8 says,

> All flesh is grass,
>> and all its beauty is like the flower of
>>> the field.
>
> The grass withers, the flower fades
>> when the breath of the LORD blows on it;
>>> surely the people are grass.
>
> The grass withers, the flower fades,
>> but the word of our God will
>>> stand forever.

We will all die of something! Cancer is just one of the means to that end. God tells us that all the days ordained for us are numbered before even one of them has come to be (Psalm 139:16). Our deaths, just like our lives, are brought about by his power and divine master plan. We have an ordained beginning ... and an end.

Surrendering Our Wills to Him

I didn't want my brother to die. I wanted him to live. But John had reached that point in spiritual maturity where he desired whatever God wanted! That's where he proved so exemplary.

He didn't kick and scream and gnash his teeth against this diagnosis. He fought it, that's true, but all along, John wanted God's will to be done. If God had chosen to cure John's cancer, he would have—and John would still be alive. The fact that God didn't heal him meant that it wasn't intended for him to live beyond those precious fifty-one years. And John was perfectly content with that. Even more, he was excited that he would meet his Savior face to face and glory in his beauty, power, and goodness.

In fact, when John received the news about his cancer, this generally shy man, who typically preferred to remain in the background, suddenly began to boldly proclaim the goodness of God in the face of adversity to anyone who would listen. He spoke in churches and civic groups, to students and teachers. He was a walking witness to everyone with whom he came into contact—from waitresses and doctors to other patients. He *lived* what he believed.

One thing I tried to do for him was to make his wait more pleasant during the hours he sat having chemo treatments. For us, this was an every Monday get-together. One of those Mondays, I was privileged to witness an unforgettable exchange between my brother and another patient.

We were waiting for an available chair in the chemo lab when a soft-spoken woman approached him. She wore a scarf around her head wrapped like a turban—a universal sign that she was a fellow cancer patient.

She said, "I don't know if you realize this or not, but we all look forward to you walking into this room every week. You're always so happy, and have such a big smile on your face. It's an amazing encouragement for the rest of us." Several other patients and their families nodded at these words.

"Why shouldn't I be happy?" he laughed. "I'm a Christian. And I know that this is all part of my Father's plan for me. He loves me and he'll get me through this—one way or the other. And either way is fine with me," he said with a grin.

The woman and several others of us in the room found ourselves fighting back tears. But my brother just smiled and said to the woman, "Thanks so much. This has been very encouraging."

She took her seat and dabbed at her eyes with a crumpled tissue. I gazed at my little brother with undisguised admiration because he wasn't faking it. He meant every word he said.

I remember a proverb that says,

> As in water face reflects face,
>   so the heart of man reflects the man.
> (Proverbs 27:19)

John's heart reflected who he was and, more importantly, whom he loved. There were times I wanted to encourage him, but each time I was the one who went away encouraged, blessed by his attitude of sweet and humble submission to the Lord.

Cancer didn't defeat John David Koon. It took his life, that's true, but he was victorious over that disease. He transcended it. And through it all, he honored his Lord by trusting in his goodness and his love.

He showed me the way. In a sense, through this book, he can show all of us the way. It's possible to honor God in the face of adversity. I've read about it in God's Word. I've seen it played out before my eyes in John's life—and in so many other lives over the decades of my nursing career. And I thank God for these memorable experiences.

How Can We Honor God through Adversity?

My goal in writing this book has not been to make anyone "feel good" about having cancer or having a loved one with it, or "feel bad" about hating it. My goal has been to come alongside you in some way and, by doing so, to help you along this journey.

However, my ultimate goal in writing this book is to glorify God. I want to proclaim Christ as the only true Savior of men and women, the only Source of true faith, and the only Solution to the problems of our lives.

It is my prayer that in this book you have found knowledge, comfort, solace, and encouragement. But there is a broader goal in all of this—that what you have been reminded of and urged to do will be applied beyond the realm of cancer to every trial in your life—now and in the future.

If we keep uppermost in our minds the importance of championing *God's* purposes for our lives, we will be able to overcome any adversity, knowing that God's will is being accomplished. Our role, as followers of Christ, is to do as Romans 12:12 commands:

> *Rejoice in hope, be patient in tribulation,*
> *be constant in prayer.*

Through every fiery struggle in our lives, we are to trust in him.

When others see this attitude shining forth through our enthusiastic acceptance of his will, we will have the opportunity to become great witnesses to the goodness of God in the face of adversity. Others will wonder, and perhaps ask, what it is that enables us to transcend the obstacles that bind others to despair. When they do, we will have the privilege of telling them where the source of our hope and faith resides—in the heart of our loving Father.

In that way, not only have we transcended our circumstances by honoring God's will for our lives, but we have also encouraged others to do the same. Comfort is a sought-after commodity when we undergo a painful trial. What a joy to take heartache and use our experience and faith to comfort others!

Praise be to God our Father and to his Son, Jesus Christ. Let me leave you with my brother's favorite verse:

May the God of hope fill you with all joy and
peace in believing, so that by the power of
the Holy Spirit you may abound in hope.
(Romans 15:13)

57

Personal Application Projects

1. List the forms of suffering that are part of
    your current situation. Be sure to include
    spiritual, emotional, or mental torment, as
    well as external, physical suffering. After each
    one, ask yourself, "How can I glorify our Lord
    through this?"

2. Read Psalm 139. Which verses do you especially
    relate to? What does this psalm teach you
    about God and his plan for your life? Compare
    what you have learned from this psalm with
    Romans 8:28–29. What is God accomplishing
    through your suffering? Is God required to tell
    us why he's doing what he's doing before we
    obey and trust him?

3. Read Psalm 46. What fears do you have? List
    them. How does knowing that God is our refuge
    and strength work to dispel these fears? What
    else do you learn about God from this psalm?

4. Read Joshua 1:5, 9. What truth brings you
    encouragement and comfort?

5. Memorize Isaiah 26:3.

6. Read Psalm 73:25–26. Is God the strength of your heart? Is he your portion forever? Are you ultimately satisfied in him? Do you resist him when he moves his hand to mold you? Write out a prayer to God that expresses your struggles and concerns, tells him that you are consciously turning to him for help, and communicates your complete trust and satisfaction in him alone. Refer to this prayer each time you find yourself suffering tribulation.

7. Read 2 Corinthians 1:3–4. What purpose does suffering serve according to this passage?

8. Read Isaiah 53. Compare this with 1 Peter 2:21–25. Describe the suffering of Jesus. How did he respond in the midst of his own suffering? Do you think he understands what you or your loved one is going through? What does Hebrews 4:15–16 encourage you to do?

9. Read Matthew 11:28–30. What is Jesus's invitation to you? What does he promise?

10. Read Hebrews 13:5–6. What promise does Jesus make here? Who is it for? Do you trust in the Lord Jesus Christ, our Savior and King?

Where Can I Get Further Help?

The following books can provide significant spiritual comfort. They may not specifically address cancer, but will help provide godly thinking through difficult times.

Bridges, Jerry, *Trusting God Even When Life Hurts* (Colorado Springs, CO: NavPress, 1988)

Howard, Deborah, *Sunsets: Reflections for Life's Final Journey* (Wheaton, IL: Crossway, 2005)

———*Where is God in All of This? Finding God's Purpose in Our Suffering* (Phillipsburg, NJ: P&R, 2009)

Lutzer, Erwin, *One Minute after You Die: A Preview of Your Final Destination* (Chicago: Moody Press, 1997)

MacArthur, John, *The Glory of Heaven: The Truth about Heaven, Angels and Eternal Life* (Wheaton, IL: Crossway, 1996)

Mack, Dr. Wayne, *Down, But Not Out: How to Get Up when Life Knocks You Down* (Phillipsburg, NJ: P&R, 2005)

———*Out of the Blues: Dealing with the Blues of Depression* (Bemidji, MN: Focus, 2006)

———*Reaching the Ear of God: Praying More—and More Like Jesus* (Phillipsburg, NJ: P&R, 2004)

———and Howard, Deborah, *It's Not Fair! Finding Hope when Times Are Tough* (Phillipsburg, NJ: P&R, 2008)

The following books and websites provide information on cancer:

Auerbach, Michael, MD, FACP, *Conversations about Cancers: A Patient's Guide to Informed Decision Making* (n.p.: Williams & Wilkins, 1996)

Buckman, Dr. Robert, *What You Really Need to Know about Cancer: A Comprehensive Guide for Patients and Their Families* (Baltimore, MD: Johns Hopkins University Press, 1997)

Eyre, Harmon J., MD, Lange, Dianne Partie, and Morris, Lois B., *Informed Decisions* (2nd edn.) (n.p.: American Cancer Society, 2001)

Fine, Judylaine, *Afraid to Ask: A Book for Families to Share about Cancer* (New York: Harper Trophy, 1996)

Morra, Marion, and Potts, Eve, *Choices: The Most Complete Sourcebook for Cancer Information* (New York: HarperCollins, 2003)

In USA

American Cancer Society: www.cancer.org

MD Anderson Cancer Center:
  epi.mdanderson.org

Tri-Cities Cancer Center: www.tccancer.org

WebMD: www.webmd.com

The Mayo Clinic: www.mayoclinic.com

In UK

Cancer Research UK: www.cancerhelp.org.uk

NHS: www.nhs.uk

Books in the *Help!* series include ...

(More titles in preparation)